COMPLETE GUIDE TO
JAW SURGERY

Essential Handbook To Techniques, Recovery
Tips, And Solutions For Corrective
Procedures, And Oral Health

DR. BRUNO HORAN

Disclaimer:

The information provided in this book, is intended for general informational purposes only and should not be considered as professional advice.

The author has made every effort to ensure the accuracy of the information presented. However, readers are advised to consult with a qualified healthcare professional before attempting any herbal remedies or making significant changes to their wellness routine. Individual health conditions vary, and what may be suitable for one person may not be appropriate for another.

It is important to note that the author is not in any endorsement deal, partnership, or affiliation with any organization, brand, or company mentioned in this book. Any references to specific products or services are based on the author's personal experience or general knowledge and do not imply an endorsement or promotion of those products or services

Contents

CONCERNING THIS BOOK

It is more important than ever to comprehend the complexities of jaw anatomy and the treatments that are related to it in the modern world when health and well-being are of the utmost importance. "Jaw Surgery: A Comprehensive Guide" explores the complex anatomy and essential operations of the jaw, illuminating the jaw's essential function in our day-to-day existence. The jaw is essential to our general health and well-being for a variety of reasons, including speaking, chewing, and face attractiveness. This book carefully examines a range of jaw conditions and their significant effects, highlighting the relationship between general systemic health and the health of the jaw.

Early detection of the telltale signs and symptoms of jaw issues can drastically change the course of treatment. This book explains the diagnostic process from the first symptoms to the use of sophisticated diagnostic techniques like CT and X-rays through in-depth case studies and professional insights. To provide readers with a proactive approach to addressing probable jaw disorders, the significance of prompt diagnosis is emphasized.

Although 'Jaw Surgery: A Comprehensive Guide' offers a beacon of clarity, navigating treatment options might be intimidating. It carefully weighs the pros and cons of non-surgical versus surgical procedures, outlining the variables that affect treatment choices and the resulting results for patients. The book provides evidence-based insights into different surgical approaches so that readers can make decisions about their health that are well-informed.

There is more to jaw surgery preparation than just the operation room. Pre-surgery measures, including dietary modifications, pharmaceutical considerations, and home preparations for the best possible recovery, are carefully outlined in this section. Pre-operative treatment is provided with a comprehensive approach by addressing stress management techniques and psychological preparedness.

On the day of surgery, anticipation gives way to reality. This section walks readers through every step of the surgical process, from hospital admission protocols to the administration of anesthetic and post-operative pain management. At a crucial stage of the therapeutic process, expectations are established and the details of the immediate post-surgery care are provided, providing comfort.

Recovery is a crucial stage where hard work and perseverance pay off. This section's main themes are accepting physical therapy, controlling discomfort, and following dietary limitations. With the help of helpful guidance on identifying potential problems and when to resume regular activities, readers can feel more confident about their recuperation process.

The road to long-term health extends beyond the moment of healing. Jaw Surgery: A Comprehensive Guide places a strong emphasis on maintaining good oral hygiene, scheduling follow-up visits, and preparing for any possible long-term consequences. Patient stories offer firsthand perspectives on life following surgery, as well as consolation and useful advice.

By directly addressing worries and fears, this section dispels myths about typical issues related to jaw surgery.

It gives readers information on possible side effects and proactive ways to reduce risks, enabling them to make wise decisions and feel at ease during treatment.

In the FAQs area, practical questions regarding visible scarring, healing times, dietary changes, and getting back to regular routines are answered with knowledge and compassion, satisfying both curiosity and clarity.

Through the provision of answers to these often-asked questions, the book acts as a reliable guide through the complexities of life after surgery.

"Jaw Surgery: A Comprehensive Guide" is an invaluable resource for anyone considering or starting the process of jaw surgery.

This book gives readers the knowledge and skills they need to make wise decisions, face recovery with confidence, and restore their general and oral health through thorough research, professional insights, and an empathetic narrative.

CHAPTER ONE

AN OVERVIEW OF JAW ANATOMY

The Jaw's Basic Structure

One of the most important parts of the skeletal structure of the human head is the jaw or mandible. The mandible, or lower jaw, and the maxilla, or upper jaw, are its two main components. The joints that unite these parts provide the movement needed for speaking, chewing, and making facial emotions. Being the only movable bone in the skull, the mandible is essential for performing functions like opening and closing the mouth.

The Jaw's Role And Significance In Everyday Activities

The jaw is a vital component of our everyday lives, enabling tasks like speaking, biting, and chewing. Beyond these fundamental functions, it also plays a major role in facial symmetry and attractiveness, which affects how we look overall.

An efficient jaw ensures that food is broken down into smaller bits that are easier to digest, which is crucial for overall health and nutrition.

Typical Jaw Conditions And Their Effects

The jaw's structure and function can be impacted by several prevalent illnesses. The common disorder known as temporomandibular joint disorder (TMJ) is characterized by discomfort and dysfunction in the muscles surrounding the jaw joint.

This disorder can seriously impair the quality of life by causing discomfort when speaking, chewing, or even just lying down.

Additional disorders include trauma-related fractures, diseases affecting the jawbone or surrounding tissues, and malocclusion (misalignment of teeth).

The Teeth And Gum Anatomy

The structure of the jaw is shaped by the teeth and gums, which are necessary for both good function and appearance.

Teeth are used for biting, ripping, and grinding food. They are an integral part of the jawbone. Supporting and shielding the roots of the teeth is the gingiva or gum tissue.

As they support appropriate nutrition and clear communication, healthy teeth and gums are essential for both oral health and general well-being.

The Impact Of Jaw Anatomy On General Health

The anatomy of the jaw is related to several facets of general health. An effective jaw enables better absorption of nutrients and assistance with digestion. Additionally, especially in cases of malocclusion or structural problems, the location of the jaw can affect respiration and even sleep patterns.

Additionally, practicing good oral hygiene—which includes routine dental examinations and taking good care of your teeth and gums—helps avoid systemic health problems like cardiovascular disease, which are linked to oral infections.

CHAPTER TWO

RECOGNIZING JAW PROBLEMS

Signs Of Jaw Disorders

Early diagnosis is essential for prompt treatment of jaw problems. Prolonged jaw pain, trouble biting or chewing, popping or clicking noises in the TMJ, and restricted jaw movement are common symptoms.

In addition, patients may have headaches, earaches, or face puffiness; these symptoms are frequently connected to problems with the jaw. Comprehending these signs facilitates timely diagnosis and therapy strategizing.

Instruments And Methods For Diagnostics

A mix of clinical examination and diagnostic testing is used to diagnose jaw problems. A comprehensive examination will be performed by the dentist or oral surgeon during the consultation to look for anomalies in range of motion, muscle discomfort, and jaw alignment. Dental X-rays are one type of diagnostic instrument that can provide thorough images of the teeth and jawbone, indicating any abnormalities in the structure or indications of arthritis.

More detailed views are provided by advanced imaging methods such as CT scans, which display the exact location of the jaw joint as well as any possible problems with the surrounding structures.

These instruments aid in the precise diagnosis of ailments such as congenital anomalies affecting the jaw, fractures, and temporomandibular joint dysfunction (TMJD).

The Use Of CT Scans And X-Rays

Because they provide images of the teeth and bones, X-rays are essential for identifying issues connected to the jaw and mouth. They are especially helpful in locating fractures, infections, or misaligned teeth that may affect the function of the jaw. On the other hand, CT scans reveal detailed pictures of the jaw's soft tissues, joints, and bones in three dimensions. When it comes to treating severe cases of TMJD, tumors, or impacted wisdom teeth, when precise anatomical information is crucial for treatment planning, this imaging technology is vital.

The Value Of Timely Diagnosis

For jaw problems to be treated less severely and to avoid consequences, early diagnosis is essential. Early detection of issues like misaligned jaws or degenerative joint illnesses allows medical professionals to prescribe the right courses of action to relieve discomfort and return normal function to the jaw.

If conditions are treated promptly, they can also stop them from getting worse and necessitate more intrusive procedures.

Case Studies of Typical Jaw Problems

Case studies highlight excellent treatment outcomes and show the variety of jaw disorders that patients may have.

For example, a patient with severe symptoms of TMJD improved dramatically when prescribed medicine and physical therapy were combined.

A further case study might present the successful use of orthodontic braces to realign a misaligned jaw, illustrating the value of early intervention in addressing developmental problems.

These illustrations stress the value of individualized treatment programs made to fit the unique jaw conditions of each patient and demonstrate the benefits of early detection and focused interventions in regaining oral health and quality of life.

CHAPTER THREE

SELECTING APPROPRIATE MEDICATION

Options For Non-Surgical Treatment

Non-surgical procedures provide the first lines of therapy and comfort for jaw problems. These may involve modifying one's way of living, such as eating differently to lessen jaw pressure or using sleep guards to ease the symptoms of teeth grinding. Additionally, jaw exercises and physical therapy can increase joint flexibility and muscular strength. These methods frequently offer substantial relief in situations of mild misalignment or transient discomfort without the need for intrusive procedures.

When No Surgery Is Required

When non-surgical treatments are ineffective at relieving symptoms or when the jaw issue is severe enough to interfere with daily activities, surgery becomes necessary. Severe discomfort, ongoing joint dysfunction, notable anatomical anomalies such as malocclusions, or a prolonged ineffectiveness of conservative measures are among the common reasons for surgery. After evaluating these variables, your healthcare professional may suggest surgery as a means of regaining function and reducing pain.

Comparing Various Surgical Methods

There are several surgical methods for jaw surgery, each suited to particular circumstances and patient requirements. Orthognathic surgery treats problems with the alignment of the jaw, whereas minimally invasive arthroscopic surgery treats diseases of the internal joints.

In cases such as micrognathia, distraction osteogenesis progressively lengthens the mandible. Comprehending these methods entails balancing variables such as duration of recuperation, intricacy, and ultimate results, directed by comprehensive discussions with your medical group.

Factors Affecting The Choice Of Treatment

Selecting the right course of treatment requires taking into account several criteria. Important factors include the patient's age, general health, the severity of the ailment, and personal preferences. While elderly patients may value shorter recovery periods, younger patients may choose procedures that permit natural growth. Making decisions is also influenced by the experience of your surgical team and your availability to specialist care, which guarantees results that are most suited to your unique situation.

Patient Outcomes And Success Rates

Patient outcomes and success rates differ based on the particular condition of the jaw and the treatment that is selected. Correcting jaw misalignment by orthodontic surgery often has a high success rate and improves bite function and facial symmetry. Compared to open surgery, arthroscopic techniques provide shorter recovery times and less scarring.

A thorough discussion of these results with your healthcare professional will enable you to make educated decisions, guaranteeing reasonable expectations and post-operative care plans for sustained success.

CHAPTER FOUR

GETTING READY FOR A JAW SURGERY

Preoperative Nutrition And Diet

Getting the correct nutrition and diet in place before having jaw surgery can have a big impact on how quickly you heal and how well you feel overall.

Make an effort to eat a diet heavy in easily digested carbohydrates and minerals.

Choose for soft foods such as soups, mashed potatoes, yogurt, and smoothies. Steer clear of chewy or hard foods like nuts, raw veggies, and rough meats that might cause jaw discomfort.

Maintaining proper hydration levels also involves drinking lots of water, limiting caffeine intake, and avoiding sugar-filled beverages.

Avoiding Medication And Supplements

It's important to discuss your current vitamins and prescriptions with your healthcare physician before jaw surgery.

Several drugs and supplements may conflict with anesthesia or raise the risk of bleeding during surgery. Blood thinners like aspirin, herbal supplements like ginkgo biloba or garlic, and certain over-the-counter painkillers are common things to stay away from. When it comes to knowing which medications to quit and when always heed the advice of your surgeon.

Getting Your House Ready For Rehab

Establishing a cozy and encouraging atmosphere at home is crucial to a successful recovery from jaw surgery.

Organize your living area to reduce the amount of reaching and bending that is required, as these actions can put strain on your jaw and impede healing.

Keep soft foods and liquids on hand, set up sleeping spaces with more cushions to prop your head up, and think about keeping necessities close at hand. Make sure all of the walkways are well-lit and unobstructed to help you avoid accidents while you're recovering.

What To Bring To The Medical Facility

Planning for your hospital stay and packing carefully for your jaw surgery will help reduce anxiety and certain you have everything you need.

Essentials include identification and insurance details, easily placed on and taken off comfortable clothing, any necessary medical records or test results, and personal hygiene products like eyeglasses and toothpaste.

Having a small bag filled with relaxing or entertaining materials, like music or books, can also help you pass the time and be comfortable.

Psychological Readiness And Stress Reduction

It's crucial to mentally and emotionally prepare for jaw surgery in addition to physically. Controlling your tension and worry can help you heal more quickly. Think about methods like meditation, deep breathing exercises, or speaking with a support group or counselor.

You can also assist reduce anxiety by talking with your healthcare provider about any worries you may have and by visualizing a successful conclusion.

Recall that it's common to experience anxiety before surgery and that managing your mental health can help make the process go more smoothly.

CHAPTER FIVE

DAY OF SURGERY

What To Anticipate On The Day Of Surgery

One of the biggest steps in bettering your general and oral health is the day of your jaw surgery. You will check in at the hospital's admissions desk upon arrival, where staff members will assist you with the last-minute arrangements.

You can anticipate a consultation with your surgical team, which will include the anesthesiologist and oral surgeon.

They will go over the process with you and address any last-minute queries you may have. Verifying information such as your medical history and any current drugs you may be taking is also a good idea at this time.

Procedure For Hospital Admissions

You will be taken to the preoperative area after being admitted, where you will change into a hospital gown. To provide you with fluids and medication both during and after the surgery, nurses will check your vital signs and start an IV line. This method makes sure you are relaxed and ready for the next step. The surgical team will double-check the details of your procedure and ensure that all required tools and equipment are available.

Pain Control And Anesthesia

To guarantee that you are comfortable and pain-free throughout jaw surgery, anesthesia is essential. You can be given intravenous sedation together with a local anesthetic to numb the surgical site, or general anesthesia, which causes a brief state of unconsciousness, depending on your particular situation.

To ensure your maximum comfort and safety, your anesthesiologist will closely monitor your vital signs and make any medication adjustments.

How Long Does The Surgery Take?

The complexity of the process determines how long jaw surgery takes. It can take anywhere from a few hours to a half day on average.

The total amount of time depends on several factors, including the extent of corrections required, whether the upper or lower jaw is involved, and any extra treatments such as bone grafts. You can be sure that throughout the procedure, your surgical team will keep you updated on developments and let you know what to anticipate.

Quick Post-Operative Care

You will be brought to the recovery room after surgery, where specially trained nurses will keep an eye on your vital signs and make sure the anesthesia wears off without a hitch. Initially, there may be some grogginess and moderate discomfort.

There will be pain management procedures in place to address any discomfort, usually with the use of oral or intravenous medicine. Instructions on post-operative care, such as how to control swelling, keep your mouth clean, and follow dietary guidelines to aid in recovery, will be given by your surgical team.

CHAPTER SIX

POST-OPTICAL REHABILITATION

Handling Soreness And Unease

Controlling pain and discomfort following jaw surgery is essential to a successful recovery. Painkillers will be recommended by your surgeon to aid with any discomfort that may arise after surgery.

To keep ahead of the pain, it's critical to take these drugs as prescribed. Furthermore, numbness and swelling in the affected area can be lessened by applying ice packs.

Make sure you adhere to your surgeon's directions regarding the frequency of ice application and the duration of each session.

Keeping oneself in a comfortable resting position can also help with discomfort management. When you're sleeping, raise your head with additional pillows to help with blood circulation and edema reduction. Steer clear of jaw-straining activities, such as eating hard food or talking too much, as these can make the healing process worse in the beginning.

Dietary Guidelines And Restrictions

Your diet will probably be limited to soft foods that don't need much chewing after jaw surgery. This facilitates healing and lessens jaw tension.

Think about eating foods high in nutrients, like smoothies, mashed potatoes, yogurt, soups, and scrambled eggs.

Steer clear of items that are firm, crunchy, or sticky since they may harm the surgery site or slow down the healing process.

Your surgeon may progressively let you resume eating more solid foods as your recuperation advances. To promote optimum healing and reduce the chance of problems, it's critical to strictly adhere to their dietary advice.

Exercises And Physical Therapy

Following surgery, physical therapy and specific exercises are important in regaining jaw strength and function.

You will be guided through specific exercises intended to enhance jaw mobility and reduce stiffness by your physical therapist or healthcare professional.

These workouts could involve resistance training with medical equipment, opening and closing exercises, and mild jaw stretches.

When doing these workouts, consistency is essential. As you feel comfortable, increase the intensity gently at first.

Throughout each session, keep in mind to stay out of your skin and pay attention to your body's cues. As your healing progresses, regular physical therapy sessions can help you restore normal jaw movement and enhance general comfort.

Signs Of Difficulties To Be Aware Of

It's critical to keep an eye out for any indications of issues that can call for medical attention during the healing phase.

If you have unusual bleeding, severe swelling, breathing or swallowing difficulties, fever, chills, or any other indicators of infection, get in touch with your doctor very away.

Keep an eye out for any changes in your bite, numbness in your face, or other strange feelings at the surgical site.

Early discovery of problems enables timely action, which can have a big impact on how well you recover.

Schedule For Getting Back To Regular Activities

The complexity of your operation and your body's healing process will determine when you can resume your regular activities. After jaw surgery, most patients can usually anticipate a gradual return to their regular activities in a few weeks to several months. But it's crucial to adhere to your surgeon's specific recovery plan and not rush the healing process.

At first, concentrate on getting enough rest and letting your body repair itself. Reintroducing employment, exercise, and social interactions should be done gradually as you get better, according to your comfort level and medical advice.

Specific instructions on when to resume particular activities and how to progressively increase your level of physical activity will be given by your surgeon.

CHAPTER SEVEN

PERMANENT COVERAGE AND MAINTENANCE

Sustaining Dental Hygiene Following Surgery

Following jaw surgery, maintaining good dental hygiene is essential for a speedy recovery and long-term health.

You should clean your mouth and teeth carefully and thoroughly, but your surgeon will give you specific recommendations based on your particular procedure. Brush your teeth carefully with a soft-bristled toothbrush and fluoride toothpaste, being sure to get all the surfaces without aggravating your healing jaw.

Using an antimicrobial mouthwash as a rinse can help lower the chance of infection. During the early healing phase, follow your surgeon's recommendations regarding any dietary restrictions or adjustments. Reintroducing meals that require more chewing should be done gradually as you make progress. Consult your surgeon for suggestions on what is appropriate according to your recovery milestones.

Check-Ins And Appointments For Follow-Up

After jaw surgery, follow-up appointments are crucial to track your healing progress and quickly treat any issues.

These consultations will be scheduled by your surgeon according to your specific recovery plan. They will examine the alignment of your jaw, look for any indications of infection or other issues, and gauge your general oral health throughout these appointments.

During these consultations, you can also talk about any persistent pain or modifications to your bite. To make sure your jaw is healing properly and to direct additional treatment, if necessary, X-rays may be obtained.

It's critical that you show up for all planned visits and that you be honest with your healthcare provider about any symptoms or problems you may be having.

Handling Prolonged Side Effects

Even while the majority of individuals recover from jaw surgery satisfactorily, some may have long-term side effects such as mild stiffness, numbness, or changes in feeling in the jaw and face.

As the nerves heal, these effects usually become better over time, but it's important to let your surgeon know if you have any ongoing issues.

It could be suggested to do jaw exercises or physical treatment to enhance jaw function and lessen stiffness.

Recuperation can be facilitated overall and adverse effects can be reduced by adhering to a balanced diet and drinking plenty of water.

Your medical staff will offer advice on how to handle any particular problems that crop up while you're recovering.

The Value Of Leading A Healthy Lifestyle

Maintaining a healthy lifestyle will help you recuperate more quickly from jaw surgery and improve your dental health in the long run.

This entails abstaining from tobacco and excessive alcohol use, maintaining an active lifestyle within the parameters specified by your rehabilitation plan, and eating a well-balanced diet high in vitamins and minerals to promote healing.

Healthy eating promotes immunological response and tissue regeneration, while consistent exercise enhances circulation and general well-being.

For the best possible recovery, stress reduction and restful sleep are also essential. By continuing these practices, you can speed up your recuperation and lower your chance of problems.

Narratives And Experiences Of Patients

While navigating your recovery, reading about other patients' experiences with jaw surgery can be reassuring and insightful.

Although every person's journey is different, learning about obstacles overcome and accomplishments can be inspiring and helpful.

Numerous patients discuss how they handle agony, maintain motivation during their recuperation, and adapt to dietary and daily schedule alterations.

Their tales frequently emphasize the value of perseverance, fortitude, and having faith in the advice of medical professionals when going through the healing process.

Knowing that healing following jaw surgery is a long process will enable you to enjoy every tiny victory and establish reasonable expectations.

Talking about your personal experiences with peers or online groups can also help you build a network of people who are understanding and sympathetic to the struggles and victories that come with this life-changing process.

CHAPTER EIGHT

COMMON ISSUES AND DIFFICULTIES

Overcoming Often Held Fears Regarding Jaw Surgery

Patients undergoing jaw surgery, commonly referred to as orthognathic surgery, may naturally have worries and anxieties.

Common concerns are the degree of discomfort and agony, how long healing will take, and whether or not the appearance of the face will alter.

It's critical to realize that anesthetic and surgical technique breakthroughs have greatly decreased pain during and after the treatment.

Your surgical team will make every effort to keep you comfortable during the procedure, including successfully controlling any discomfort afterward.

How long the recuperation takes is another issue. Although every patient's recuperation period may differ due to the intricacy of the procedure and personal healing variables, your surgeon will offer a precise schedule and instructions for aftercare. Carefully adhering to these guidelines can facilitate a quicker recovery.

A change in the way your face looks can also be concerning. Orthognathic surgery can improve face harmony without significantly changing appearance by addressing functional problems such as bite alignment and chewing difficulties.

Your surgeon will go over the anticipated results in advance with you to make sure you have reasonable expectations and to address any worries you may have regarding changes to the appearance of your face.

Possible Issues And How To Handle Them

The dangers and problems of jaw surgery are the same as those of any surgical operation. Bleeding, infection, nerve damage, and momentary or infrequently permanent changes in sensation or movement are a few examples of these. With meticulous planning, exact surgical methods, and postoperative monitoring, your surgical team is trained to reduce these risks to the lowest possible level.

The management of bleeding during or following surgery involves the use of precise surgical techniques and post-operative monitoring.

Even though they are uncommon, infections are usually avoided by using antibiotics and sterile surgical techniques. Nerve injuries are rare but can result in temporary numbness or tingling. Following surgery, they are closely monitored to ensure a progressive return of sensation.

Long-Term Impacts And Coping Strategies

Planning and recuperation from jaw surgery require an understanding of the long-term repercussions. The short-term effects, such as better bite function and face symmetry, should go away in a few weeks or months, but the long-term advantages can greatly improve the quality of life. Along with going over these advantages, your surgeon will offer advice on how to handle any lingering discomfort while you heal.

When To Get Medical Advice

For the best possible outcome following surgery, it is crucial to understand when to consult a doctor. If you have significant pain that does not go away after taking prescribed medicine, excessive bleeding, fever, growing redness and swelling, symptoms of infection, or any sudden changes in movement or sensation in your face, get in touch with your surgeon right once.

Mental And Emotional Assistance

Having jaw surgery may affect one's mental and emotional health. It's common to feel a range of emotions, such as enthusiasm about the expected outcomes or even dissatisfaction or dread.

Getting help from friends, family, or a professional can help you deal with these feelings. To help you connect with others who have had similar surgeries, your surgical team may also provide resources or links to support groups. These connections can be quite helpful in offering emotional support along your journey.

CHAPTER NINE

FREQUENTLY ASKED QUESTIONS ABOUT JAW SURGERY

How Much Time Does It Take To Recover?

The length of recovery following jaw surgery varies based on the intricacy of the operation and the healing rates of the individual.

The first healing period usually lasts between six and eight weeks, during which time pain and swelling gradually go down. Patients are usually instructed to adhere to a stringent post-operative care plan, which includes maintaining a stable jaw and doing as directed by their doctors for pain management.

It may take several months to fully recover, at which point comfort and normal jaw function return. To guarantee a seamless recuperation, your surgeon will offer personalized instructions based on your particular circumstances.

Will The Scars Show Up?

The goal of contemporary jaw surgery methods is to reduce noticeable scars. To lessen visibility, incisions are carefully made inside the mouth or along the wrinkles in the skin.

External incisions may be required for some operations, especially those affecting the chin or jawline, although they are carefully planned to provide the best possible cosmetic results.

It's crucial to talk to your surgeon about any scarring issues you may have during the pre-operative consultations. They may offer particular advice based on the operation you'll be having.

What Kind Of Eating Plan Must I Adhere To?

It is usually advised to start with a soft or liquid diet after jaw surgery to give the jaw room to recover naturally. Smoothies, soups, mashed potatoes, and protein shakes can all fall under this category. You can progressively move on to more solid foods as your jaw heals and functions better. Hard, crunchy, or sticky foods must be avoided in the early phases of recovery to minimize discomfort and potential injury to the healing tissues. You may receive a comprehensive meal plan from your surgeon or a dietitian, customized to your unique requirements and healing process.

When Can I Go Back To Work Or School?

The type of treatment done, each person's rate of recovery, and the physical demands of your job or school activities all play a role in when you should return to work or school following jaw surgery. Typically, patients should plan to take a week or two off from work or school to concentrate on their initial healing.

For the best healing during this period, relaxation and adherence to post-operative care guidelines are essential. When it's safe to return to your regular activities after surgery, your surgeon will give you advice based on your recovery status and any applicable restrictions.

How Can I Guarantee The Greatest Result?

You must actively participate in your pre-operative care and post-operative rehabilitation to receive the greatest result from jaw surgery. Talk to your surgeon in-depth about your expectations, worries, and medical history before surgery.

Pay close attention to all pre-operative instructions; these may involve changing your medication schedule or way of life.

Following surgery, carefully follow your surgeon's instructions regarding your food, amount of physical activity, rest, and dental cleanliness. Keep track of your healing progress and swiftly address any concerns by attending any follow-up appointments.

You may greatly increase the chance that your jaw surgery will go well by keeping lines of communication open with your medical team and carefully following their instructions.

To ensure that patients feel informed and ready for their surgical journey, these responses are intended to address common questions about jaw surgery and offer clarity and helpful counsel.